Here are 5 rules health must follow...

I LOVE YOU JENNIFER AND MAKENZIE!!

HEALTH IS PRACTICALLY FREE

Don't Wait Until it Costs You Everything
John Fresh, D.C.

Table of Contents:

An interactive guide to great articles and research for better health.   60

Introduction

Health needs no introduction. We all want it, even if we define it or want to enjoy it differently. The one thing we can agree on is that no one wants to lose their health. In fact, people want to be as healthy as they can be. However, many times we want health by living however we choose. Unfortunately often many of those choices do not follow the rules of health.

Health is not a mystery, the mystery is why do we continue to try and find health in places it does not exist? How we live our lives is our best opportunity to have the greatest impact on our health. The truth is that there are proven methods that support how the body is designed to function and better health is always the result. (Ref: Health Articles and Research: INTRODUCTION #1: 10 Ways To Live Longer (Mercola.com)). Actually, the bodys' natural state is health. Every function it performs is designed to meet the needs of every cell, in conjunction with meeting the needs of trillions of other cells, tissues, organs, and organ systems in a united effort to promote, healing and health.

There are 2 main ways people learn about health. The first and best way is when they are taught about health from others. Preferably before they have health concerns. Second, usually occurs after they have a health concern or scare. Once a person has lost some aspect of their health they'll be more likely to do whatever it takes to get it back. This is when the motivation to get healthy is at its peak. In many situations poor health is what seems to get people's attention the most. However, these concerns can be short lived once their symptoms have resolved. What usually occurs is that people restore just enough health to shut off the "symptom alarm" before they get back to their busy lives. Which is a concern because in most cases these health problems occurred from neglecting one or more of the 5 foundations of health. This won't usually happen over night, most health problems progress over time. So, one of the greatest dangers to a person's health and quality of life occurs once symptoms have gone away. They go back to the lifestyle that caused the health crisis, while never addressing the poor lifestyle habits that caused them. Now, the next time these symptoms appear the underlying health issue has usually progressed. Unfortunately diagnostic test reveal this to be the case for many people who address their health by symptoms alone.

So, once you have addressed your symptoms and completed any necessary emergency care, it's time to get to work and find out which foundational principle of health has been neglected. The symptoms are a clue to where you body is asking for health. We should be motivated to determine the cause of that symptom. This will help to provide our body with whatever it needs to heal and repair itself. It can even provide us with the information we need to take our health to the next level. Just like how a tight muscle is a symptoms of a muscle that needs to be stretched or how being thirsty is a symptom that we need more water. However, if we continue to deny what the body is asking for, things will get worse, even if the symptoms temporarily go away.

Thank God we have a body that can communicate its needs to us. The better we listen and meet those needs, the better our health. The only thing better is to know what the body requires before it even has to ask! Guess what, for the most part we do!!! So, it is important that we are proactive. We need to help ourselves by continually learning more about how to apply the 5 Foundations of Health. Because if we miss out on any one of these foundational principles it is impossible to experience your full health potential throughout your lifetime. We need to apply all 5 principles to be at our best.

The 5 Foundations of Health are 1. LIFE 2. INTAKE 3.MOVEMENT 4. REST and 5. POSITIVITY. We are going to take the time to go through each of these foundational principles in the following chapters. Here is an extremely brief look at each of the 5 foundational principles of health. Life, represents the impulses that animate all living tissue, keeping them alive. Intake is what we eat and drink and the impact that has on health and disease. Movement is essential for the brain and the body to be healthy and strong. Rest is when our body receives the majority of our healing and repair. Positivity is an intentional way of thinking about and filtering our experiences which will determine how we see the world and most importantly how we respond to it.

What makes something a foundational principle for health? That's pretty simple. If no matter who you are, what condition you have, and regardless of your age, if you apply these foundational truths your health will improve. Next, these principles should not only produce better health for every person, every time, these benefits should also be repeatable. This is what makes Life, Intake, Movement, Rest, and Positivity foundational principles for health. These 5 foundational principles have been proven to provide better health for centuries.

What does NOT make the list of foundational principles for health. Methods that would, over time, make a healthy person sick. This in a nutshell is the problem with trying to use emergency care for health care. Emergency care, drugs, surgery, injections, pain killing, and so on, focus on doing whatever it takes to treat symptoms or damage, usually caused by poor habits. This is obviously excluding sudden traumatic events. Emergency care may do a good job at relieving symptoms or addressing damage that has become more dangerous than the negative impact of the emergency care itself. But, it is important to know that there is a cost to prolonged use of emergency care as health care, especially when talking about prolonged medication use. However, in this context I am specifically talking about conditions that were caused by lifestyle and have a lifestyle solution. Which most health problems do fall into that category. You will find that there is a lot of research that will support the fact that over 85 % of chronic diseases are preventable. So, for this large group of people prolonged emergency care, without a change in lifestyle, will cost them their health. In the end emergency care would make a healthy person sick, not healthier. So, how could it ever make a sick person healthy?

I feel like I need to mention that this does not include people who have been born or developed a need to utilize the marvels of modern medicine. This is not about a person born a diabetic. Even those these principles can help that person achieve better health, this conversation is more about the person who becomes diabetic through lifestyle choices. Ok, having said all that, this is not a book about the wonderful emergency procedures that we do have in place for emergency situations. This book is about the foundational principles required for anyone and everyone to achieve better health.

So, the simple question to ask yourself, for treating the cause of health issues, and planning a long term solution to restore and improve health is...would living this way make a healthy person healthier. How about if they lived this way for 1, 5, or 10 years? How about if they lived like this for the rest of their life? If yes, they would be healthier, it's probably worth considering the benefits for you and your family. Chances are they are connected in some way to these 5 principles. If no, the best place to start would be with these 5 foundational principles. You don't have to start by doing everything perfect, you start by doing a little better each day. Focus on progress. In most cases, in a relatively short period of time you will restore the health you had lost or build on the health you have been enjoying. Fortunately, better health, not always perfect health, is the result...every time. Unfortunately, no one can guarantee you perfect health, even if you are doing everything correctly. There are just things we do not control. So even though perfect health involves some things we do not control, better health is always under our control.

I had asked the lord to give me something unique, that people needed, based on the gifts and talents he had given me. In the middle of the night I woke up and for 2 hours kept putting down some initial thoughts about the next thing he wanted me to do. This book is the story of that journey and my dependence on Jesus to serve him and others in his name.

Chapter 1

Life

The power that made us, heals and repairs us, and meets all the needs of our body each and every day.

This power, called LIFE, travels over the brain and nerves, through the spine to each and every cell. These cells are the building blocks that make up our body. The brain, nerve, spine, and cell relationship is the most important, yet most overlooked and under cared for foundational aspect of our health. (Ref: Chapter: Health Articles and Research: LIFE #1: The Nervous System In 9 Minutes (CTE Skills.com on YouTube)). That sentence was a mouthful, but I hope I found a way to say it all. Inflammation, irritation, stretching, compressing a nerve or anything else that will alter the already perfect spark of life from the brain to the cells will always lead to weaker cell. Weaker cells ultimately lead to less health.

If you would allow me, I would like to make an analogy. Think of the messages from the brain to the cells like a guitar that is in tune, making the perfect "tone" or sound to the listener. Tone, /tōn/, noun: a musical or vocal sound with reference to its pitch, quality, and strength. In this analogy, the brain is the guitar player, the nerves are the cords, the spine is the guitar, and your eardrums are the cells. The right sound at the right time, for the right amount of time is pleasing to the ear. Achieving the perfect tone making beautiful music possible. The beautiful music represents health. It is important to remember that we have trillions of instruments, cells, in our orchestra which create beautiful music or health for our whole body each and every day. So, the brain and nerve system is not just playing all the instruments individually, they are also the conductor.

So, what could possibly disrupt this beautiful symphony of health? I will save the discussions about intake (nutrition), movement, rest, and positivity until their appropriate sections. However, what fits perfectly in this section is the path the brain and nerves take to get to the cells of the body. The spine and the joints of the spine protects the brain and nerves. These carry the vital information or sparks of life the brain and nerves transmit to each and every cell. (Ref: Chapter: Health Articles and Research: LIFE #2: Structure Of The Vertebral Column - Functions Of The Spine - Bones Of The Vertebrae (Whats Up Dude on YouTube)). You could also think of the spine as a hose that protects and guides water to a garden. The faucet where all the water comes out represents the skull that holds the brain. The hose that carries the water is like the spine carrying the nerves, nerve impulses, and messages from the brain to the body. The garden is like the cells that require the messages from the brain to survive and thrive. The condition or health of the hose can change the flow of water to the garden. In the same way the health of the spine affects the flow of life to the cells. A healthy hose or spine means a healthy garden or cells. An unhealthy hose, like a hose with a kink, can limit the amount of water getting to the garden. This would mean the garden is getting less water than it needs to flourish. In this analogy the garden may wilt or not produce as much fruit, especially when under conditions of extreme stress. The more stress in an environment, the faster deficiencies and weaknesses will be exposed. Unfortunately, this is also true for us. An unhealthy spine causes less life to get to the cells, which ultimately cause our health to suffer in any number of ways. The list of ways our health can be affected from this one problem, the spine irritating and changing the life impulses to the cells, is hard to measure. The reason being is that the impulses of life that flow over our nerves and through our spines control and coordinate everything our bodies do.

Now, we have been taught how to take care of so many areas of our body. Like how our heart and lungs require cardiovascular exercise. How our muscles need movement to promote strength and flexibility. We are even taught how to take care of our teeth by brushing them regularly. The question is, how well have you been taught to know when your posture is off track or how to take care of the joints of your spine? In order to keep your spine healthy. Have you been taught how to tell which joints are stuck or kinked and how to get them moving again? Stuck joints are a huge problem because they begin the process of degeneration by causing inflammation. So, these stuck joints over time lead to arthritis, disc disease, and nerve irritation. The process of getting arthritis and disc disease from a stuck joint begins within 2 weeks from the joint being stuck. Stuck joints can occur by doing little things improperly over time or with big things like a sudden fall or trauma. Stuck joints turn into subluxated joints, which means the stuck joint is not only causing inflammation that leads to arthritis and disc disease, but is changing the impulses or sparks of life from the brain to the cells. Subluxations cause abnormal nerve impulses and since nerve impulses determine the health of a cell, the abnormal impulse causes abnormal or weaker cells. This ultimately means less health for the entire body.

There is a normal process in the body, called autophagy, where older cells are replaced by newer cells. This ultimately is how health and disease occur over time. It is pretty simple, healthy nerve impulses make healthy cells and unhealthy nerve impulses make unhealthy cells. With unhealthy nerve impulses the cells continue to get weaker and the body becomes more vulnerable to disease. On the other hand, with healthy nerve impulses cells get stronger and the body gets stronger. The whole person becomes healthier and better able to resist disease. The strength and health of cells determine the strength and health of a person. So, keeping spinal joints moving and aligned is one of our foundational responsibilities. Improving spinal health will minimize and prevent subluxations while simultaneously supporting the brain, nerves, spine, cells, and overall health. There is a sound scientific reason it has such a great impact on each person's overall health. Which is, regardless of what health problems any person is going through, by taking care of the joints of the spine you are promoting better health for the brain and nerve system. The brain and nerve system make up the master control system, the system that knows exactly how to meet the needs of each and every cell in the body. The brain and nerve system travel through the spine for protection, so our ability to care for our spine not only determines how well the brain and nerve system is protected but how well it works. This in my opinion makes the health of our brain, nerve system, and spine as important and possibly even more important than all the other organs and systems that is controls. But we don't have to decide which systems is the most important. We need to take care of them all.

One last thing, there are many parts of your body that can be replaced. But, we want to make sure we are doing everything possible to make our original parts last as long as possible. There is nothing better than our original custom made parts. So, to make that possible we need to look at what history has taught us. Which parts wear out the most and cause the most suffering? We know the most worn out parts of most people's body over time and the number one cause of chronic pain and suffering is joint problems. Specifically the joints of the spine. These joint problems don't usually happen overnight, they happen over a lifetime. Usually while people have very little or no idea it is happening. What happens to people with undiagnosed and untreated spinal joint problems? Spinal joint problems irritate the nerves causing pain and suffering. Stopping people from living their lives. Sometimes the pain will go away and people will get back to their lives, but that does not always mean that health was restored to their spinal joint problem. As a result, the degeneration in the spinal joint progresses until their next episode of muscle and/or nerve irritation. That is why I say undiagnosed and untreated, because many times people will get something for the pain, inflammation, or muscle spasms, but not the joint problem. In many cases the joint problem is the underlying problem. Posing the greatest risk to your health and quality of life.

Here is proof that spinal problems are a threat to our health and quality of life. If you were to study the progression of joint problems in the spine, you will find that too many go undiagnosed and untreated. As a result, this leads to spinal problems progressing as people age. Many of these problems could have been avoided if they were addressed closer to when the joint injury first occurred. Here are the facts. There are 20% of teens who have mild disc degeneration without symptoms. By the time a person is 70 years old 60% of discs are severely degenerated with or without symptoms (Urban and Roberts 2003). When looking at the last lumbar disc in the spine, the L5-S1 disc of 70-year olds, you will find over 90% have been degenerated (Hagiwara et al. 2014).

If we were to look at people with zero back pain, no symptoms, 64% would have abnormal discs. Of that 64%, 52% had disc bulges, 27% disc protrusions, and 1% disc extrusions. While 38% of individuals have abnormalities at multiple disc levels (Jensen et al. 1994). "The prevalence of disk degeneration in asymptomatic individuals increased from 37% of 20-year-old individuals to 96% of 80-year-old individuals. Disk bulge prevalence increased from 30% of those 20 years of age to 84% of those 80 years of age. Disk protrusion prevalence increased from 29% of those 20 years of age to 43% of those 80 years of age. The prevalence of annular fissure increased from 19% of those 20 years of age to 29% of those 80 years of age." (Brinjinkji et al. 2015). When looking at how many people have arthritis at 18-44 years of age, there is around 7%. In the group that was 65 or older, the percentage of people with arthritis went up 43% to 50% (2010-2012 NHIS). I want to thank Bret Contreas for putting together the article which included the research I was looking for on the internet concerning the progression of spinal disease with age (https://bretcontreras.com/degeneration-more-like-normal-aging/).

I always like to focus on what we do control concerning our health. I have the same philosophy concerning spinal health This approach has helped a lot of people get their life back. Some people even say they haven't felt this young or been able to do the things they are able to do now in years. Because of the success we have had with so many people, I have a different approach on how to use this data. My experience looking at thousands of x-rays shows that not everyone's spine ages the same and neither do the individual joints of the same spine. How we perform the activities of our day do determine the amount of wear and tear on a spine. Like a car driving out of alignment and the tires wearing out faster on the edges. Most importantly I have seen how taking care of the spine has improved posture, removed nerve irritation, and restored motion to the stuck joints of the spine. Also, showing people how to reduce stress on their spine has allowed them to perform their daily activities longer and stronger with less irritation to the spine.

So this spinal damage that so many people have is not necessarily normal aging alone! It is just very common. Why, because we have not been taught how to take care of the joints of our spine throughout our lifetime. In those same spines that you see arthritis in a person that is 80 years old, you will also see joints that look 10 or 20 years old. Aren't all the joints the same age? Why do they look different? It is because healthy joints age normally. Unhealthy joints, like stuck joints, age faster. That is also why in a younger person with unhealthy joints, you can see joints that are much older than their chronological age. If it was normal aging all the joints would age similar to the persons age. But, this is usually never the case! Stuck joints, a joint that is not moving normally or is out of alignment, increase the rate at which spinal joints age. They can occur from things like your body not adapting to falling 5000 times learning how to walk. How you sleep, sit in chairs, watch tv, and look at your phone. What sports or activities you were involved in growing up. Have you had any falls on the playground, riding your bike, or running and playing with friends. The list goes on concerning moments that cause stuck joints and misalignment that if not addressed cause spinal health to decline with time in those areas.

While a perfect spine may not be obtainable, the healthiest version of the spine you have will prevent stuck or injured joints from aging faster. This will have an incredible impact on your health through every age and stage of life. What do you think a person's teeth would be like if they ate harmful things for the teeth and never took care of them. Answer: a lot worse than someone who did take care of them throughout their lifetime. The same rules apply to the health of your spine and discs..

Now, many people will be proactive and begin to work on restoring muscle flexibility and core strength, which is great! But alone does not address joint problems. While muscle health is important, restoring health to the joint that has a problem and muscle health will have the greatest impact. Joint problems become most evident when we look at imaging. People can clearly see the different characteristics of a healthy versus an unhealthy joint. When you put up a person's x-rays or MRI of their spine you are looking at the changes to the joints caused by stuck or subluxated joints. Now, it is always important to make the core or outside stronger to protect the inside or spine better. However, it is just as important to take care of the inside or spine too. So, if you have spine, disc, or joint problems taking care of the core alone will not completely address the health of the joints and discs of your spine.

This is important to remember because you only get one brain, nerve system, and spine. How you take care of this aspect of your health will impact every area of your life. The sooner you learn how to take care of it the better. Taking care of the spine is necessary for brain, nerve, and cell health. Of course under the topic of intake (nutrition) we could talk for days on the different ways to keep the brain, nerves, and cells healthy, but there are already a ton of books on that subject. However, this book is focused on what is not being addressed, which is the impact that spinal joint health can have on your overall health, wellbeing, and active lifestyle. I hope I was able to encourage you to consider the value of making spinal health a priority for you and your family. On one hand I am concerned about the cost of not communicating the devastating effects that poor spinal health can have on every area of your life. I would hope that you understand the influence it has on the LIFE force that your spine protects, well enough, for you to make any necessary changes or additions to your spinal care. On the other hand I am excited about the incredible life that I know and have seen is waiting for you when you make spinal joint health a priority. I have seen and cared for enough spines to know how a person's health is impacted for the better. Sometimes within just weeks of taking better care of the joints of their spine. I am amazed at how people who have had all types of aches and pains for 10, 20, 30, 40, and even 50 years and beyond have responded to restoring joint health, and in turn LIFE to the body, through chiropractic care. Many of these people have been everywhere and tried everything. Everything except restoring health to the joints of their spine, which then restored health to the nerves that were causing the pain. (Ref: Chapter: Health Articles and Research: LIFE #3: Stiffness And pain In The Morning And After Activity (FreshStartChiro1 on YouTube)). The first step is being evaluated by a chiropractor. A chiropractor is the one professional that specializes in joint health and spinal care. They will be able to help you analyze the joints of your spine and restore health to stuck or subluxated joints.

Foundational Habits…

Life happens through joint health. The spine is made of bones and discs that are only millimeters away from the tissues of the brain and nerves that carry LIFE to the body. Taking care of our spine is one of our greatest responsibilities. Keep your spine as healthy as possible to keep your brain, nerves, and cells healthy. These are the building blocks to a healthy, happy, independent, and active life.

Chapter 2

Intake

The air we breathe, the water we drink, and the foods we put into our body.

I could probably stop right there. Most of the time when it comes to our intake, it is more of a discipline issue, than it is about knowing what we should and shouldn't be drinking or eating. Here is the easiest way to determine if you are making healthy choices. If it comes from the earth it is probably the best drink and food choice you can make towards better health. This has been proven to be true in the case of water. It is also true concerning the best food choices that are available. The best foods are whole foods. So, we should eat them in their whole food form, in a variety of shapes and colors. A variety of whole foods provides us with an array of essential nutrients. We would not be able to obtain all these nutrients with a limited diet. These are nutrients are body requires, that is why they are named essential. Because our bodies can not make certain nutrients from other building blocks or foods. The body has to get essential nutrients from whole foods that have them or supplementation. Once again whole foods are always better. But, if you have a limited selection of whole foods that you eat, you may want to consider supplementation. Unfortunately, there is a problem. Water and foods that are healthy are being negatively affected by a number of factors. Practices of farming, genetically engineered food, sprays to keep pests off, and techniques to create bigger and more abundant crops with a higher yield are harming our water and food supplies. However, what is most important is that we are aware of these practices. This allows us to choose healthy water and food that is brought to us in healthy ways.

Let's talk about water. Water is the best thing you can drink, however, water from the tap is not being monitored properly. The infrastructure to carry the water is declining and the levels of harmful chemicals in the water are rising. These problems are and not being reported to the public. Considering these factors makes filtering your water a necessity. (Ref: Health Articles and Research: INTAKE #1: Water Poisoning Alerts Hidden From Public (Mercola.com)). This article from Dr. Mercola that was referenced above points out the dangers of the water we may be drinking. It also offers solutions and explains the different filtering systems you have to choose from to ensure you are drinking healthy water. The better the water you drink the better it pulls toxins out of your body creating a detoxifying effect. On the other hand bad water sources can deposit toxins into your body. Alkaline water from specific filter systems can even contribute to creating a healthier more alkaline environment inside your body. Hydration is a vital need of the body for health. There is nothing that hydrates better than healthy water.

The quality of the air we breathe, especially in public places or outdoors spaces is sometimes hard for us to control. Let's look at some ways we can improve the air we breathe. In our homes we can keep up with the filters and vents by having a yearly plan to change old filters and clean the vents. They are the lungs of the house and workplace. It is very important that we keep our houses dry and use dehumidifiers if necessary. The reason being is that humidity and moisture can produce mold, which has a negative impact on health. Many times mold problems can go undiagnosed and untreated Unsuspecting people may be treated for other health conditions that present similar symptoms as mold. If you suspect mold in your home there are kits you can buy to determine if you have a mold problem.

Whenever you do have a decent air supply available remember to breathe deeply and often. Intake of air, deep breathing, has a number of health benefits. Positively impacting people's health mentally, physically, and spiritually with zero negative side effects. The lungs expand and more oxygen enters the body. Neurologically, deep breathing promotes rest and relaxation by minimizing the "stress" response. Breath is the foundation of many practices that clear and calm the mind and body. There are a number of different breathing techniques you can try. There are even exercise programs that focus on breath.

So, why don't people breath deeply more often, it's free, you can do it anywhere and at any time? The answer is that we all just forget to take deep breaths. Usually when we or someone else reminds us to take a breath we can feel the difference almost immediately. So, it is beneficial to get in the habit of practicing deep breathing. A great way to do that is to set reminders and strategically place cues in plain view to encourage and remind you to breathe deeply.

When it comes to food, I believe that God makes everything perfect. However, when the food we eat is fed unhealthy nutrition or water, exposed to unhealthy toxins, either in the way it is farmed, stored, or transported it is a step in the wrong direction. This can turn what started out to be a healthy food into an unhealthy food. Unhealthy foods cause people that eat them to become unhealthy. The change from healthy to unhealthy may not become apparent right away. However time always reveals the cost poor choices have on our health. Anymore it is not good enough just to eat healthy foods, we have to take the additional time to find out how it made it to our tables. (Ref: Health Articles and Research: INTAKE #2: What makes most foods so dangerous, even "healthy foods" (Mercola.com)).

It is not my specialty to discuss the impact of losing biodiversity by growing the same crops over and over, while not giving the land time to replenish its nutrients. I believe many times we are all a step behind in understanding nature and the cycles it follows. God's ways are beyond human comprehension or understanding. Even our best explanations are amended as we gather new information as life and experiences provide. If there is one method of determining the best choices for eating and drinking is to keep it simple. Don't let all the articles, research, or marketing confuse you. Here is what to consider when thinking about which choices promote health and pass the test of time. Remember this golden rule to get you started. If it comes from the earth, is grown, and delivered responsibly it will be better for your health. Another simple or foundational rule involves eating a variety of healthy foods to get the different nutrients the body requires. It is also important to avoid sugars and unhealthy grains that promote inflammation, cause insulin sensitivity, and metabolic diseases. (Ref: Health Articles and Research: INTAKE #3: The Truth About Sugar Addiction (Mercola.com)).

The most health benefits have been shown to involve food choices that include fruits, vegetables, healthy fats, and protein. The numbers and sources of what to eat and when to eat vary from person to person and can require blood work and other testing. When to eat, including fasting and intermittent fasting, has been shown to have a positive impact on health all the way down to the health of the cells. This however is another area that differs for each person.

When we talk about food in a package, that's when things get complicated. The labels are difficult to read. Once we figure out what the words mean and how those ingredients negatively impact our health, they change the name or find another ingredient that we and our body does not recognize. While the back of the package may be hard to read, the front of the package can be even more deceiving. There is a difference between healthy food and marketing that a food is healthy. Many companies may claim their product promotes a health benefit based on the benefits of a specific ingredient. If you are looking to receive the full health benefit from any ingredient, you are usually much better off consuming the ingredient from nature than the processed version. This processed version is usually put in a box with a list of other products that have very little or even zero health benefits. Remember in a natural environment, foods have their greatest health benefits. In nature these foods are already packaged with all the additional nutrients they require to maximize their health benefits. There are so many benefits to intaking our food from nature. Many are known, but there are still many benefits that are unknown to us at this time.

However, what manufacturers will do is process that healthy food until it does not even resemble or have the benefits of that food in nature. This strips the food of all the other vital components as if mining for what the company or food label values as gold. But it can be fool's gold. This is not to say we can't all enjoy these products or how easy they are to grab in a pinch when we are on the go. However, processed foods should not be the foundation of our diet. Over time these products alone create unhealthy environments in the body increasing a person's risk for a number of different health concerns. Whatever the environment is on the inside of a person will eventually be what is expressed on the outside. This healthy or unhealthy environment will spill over into that person's state of health and quality of life. I will just give you one example of the devastating impact of marketing.

"Fat free" was a claim that many marketers used to influence customers who were looking to reduce fat intake and lose weight. They were leading people to think that fat made people overweight. This was a huge mistake. First, there are different types of fat and it is important to know our brain , nerves, hormones, and the cell walls of our body, just to name a few things, are made of fat. They must have good fats to build and even repair these structures on a daily basis. We need good fats to be healthy! This "fat free" marketing campaign stopped people from consuming the healthy fats our body's need and started people consuming processed unhealthy "fat free" foods. Research has shown that many of these "fat free" products have led to inflammation in the body creating an unhealthy acidic environment. Foods that cause inflammation and these acidic environments contribute to diseases like diabetes, heart disease, cancer, and other metabolic diseases. Conversely, solutions to many of today's health issues include removing harmful sugars and unhealthy grains to help reduce inflammation and acidity in the body. Inflammation also oxidizes cholesterol, making it unhealthy, causing it to stick to arteries that sugar and inflammation has damaged. Cholesterol, which is one type of fat, has many important roles it plays in our body. Healthy cholesterol is vital to each and every person. Healthy cholesterol does not stick to artery walls, like unhealthy cholesterol. The "fat free" movement never solved the problem it was created to address, weight loss, and ended up causing a number of other health problems and metabolic disorders in the process.

Omega 3 fats are one of the healthy fats that we need to have in our body. You can find high amounts of Omega 3 fats from fatty fish, algae, and several high fat plant foods. Omega 3 fats even make healthier more pliable cell walls for all the cells in our body. So, having Omega 3 in our body is good, but problems can occur involving inflammation when we have an imbalance in the amounts or ratio of Omega 6 to Omega 3 in our body. This happens from eating too many foods that are high in unhealthy Omega 6 fats like processed snacks, fast foods, cakes, fatty meats, and cured meats, while not eating enough healthy Omega 3 fats. The greater the ratio, of Omega 6 being higher than Omega 3, the more inflammation and the more diseases that are associated with that inflammation. The closer the ratio of Omega 6 to Omega 3 is to 1:1 the better. However you are still considered in a healthy range when the ratio is 4 (Omega 6):1 (Omega 3). You can find out your numbers with a blood test and retest when you want to monitor how your numbers are improving. This is a great way to determine the levels of inflammation currently in your body and how you can use dietary changes and supplements to improve the Omega 6 to Omega 3 ratio and reduce inflammation. When considering your health this is vitally important because inflammation is practically the cause or at least involved in almost every disease process.

Now at this point, I know you know that whole food is the best source for all nutrients. However there may be a reason that you do not have a balanced diet to provide you with everything your body needs to be healthy. Here are some supplements to consider to help meet your body's basic nutritional requirements. Your needs may go beyond what you are getting from food alone. These basic supplements can help you get the most from the food you eat and ensure you have all the essential vitamins and minerals your body requires. Creating a healthy environment in your gut for digesting food. This healthy environment will improve your immune system and reduce inflammation. Supplements will fill in any gaps and provide your diet with the building blocks for a healthy brain, nerves, and cells.

These supplements are what I would call the core 4. The core 4 includes a (1) multivitamin, (2) omega 3, (3) probiotics, and (4) digestive enzymes. I call them the core 4 because I have heard these supplements talked about from two of my most reliable resources for many years and they still have their full support. Over the years I have heard them talked about in seminars and now they are talked about by practically everyone. They are the most basic supplements that benefit each and every person. However, some people do require additional specific supplements to meet their unique needs. So, it is always good to check with your doctor and pharmacist to make sure you choose what's best for you. Especially if you are taking any other supplements or medication that may interact inappropriately. We want everyone to be on the same page when it comes to our health.

The reason the core 4 are so important and fiber for that matter is because they make it possible for the body to perform all its functions better. One major thing they do is aid in assimilation and digestion of all the foods we eat. This will ultimately further benefit all other healthy nutritional choices by providing a healthy digestive system. The core 4 allows us to get more nutrition from the foods we eat, while also being better able to utilize those materials to build a healthier body. The core 4 is also able to help the body to better perform many of its other required functions for health as well. Multivitamins provide the keys that are required to to turn on and off many of the reactions inside cells. These reactions are what make practically everything in our body work at the most fundamental levels. Healthy fats make up the brain, the cells of our body, and are the foundational components for many things in our body, like hormones. So, this is why healthy fats make the list. The one thing you may also want to investigate is the source that the supplement comes from, like fish or shellfish in the case of omega 3's. Especially if you have any allergies, food sensitivities or dietary restrictions. There are usually alternatives for each person, like for Omega 3's there is also a vegan alternative. The "good" bacteria of the gut, which the probiotics support plays a major role in digestion and the immune system as well. An imbalance in the bacteria of the gut can cause inflammation, leaky gut, and a number of other health issues. (Ref: Health Articles and Research: INTAKE #4: How Gut Bacteria Influence Your Metabolism (Mercola.com)). The enzymes help food to be more easily broken down into nutrients that are brought into the body for use by the cells. Fiber is important because it feeds the good bacteria in the gut, helps better control sugar, and can be filling to protect you from unnecessary calories. Like I mentioned before, I have found these basic nutritional tools by following people and resources I trust for years. Their recommendations and the research that they have gathered promoting these products and their health benefits in our diet have only been confirmed over time.

There are many other vital supplements that are required by a number of processes in the body and there are too many to list. There are specific tests that use blood work, saliva, and stool to help determine your specific needs. There is one more important thing I will mention, which is the importance of monitoring your vitamin D levels. Vitamin D has such a big influence on so many areas of our health. Here is a great resource concerning vitamin D. (Ref: Health Articles and Research: INTAKE #5: Vitamin D Resource Page (Mercola.com)). It is important to note that if there is a health benefit of a specific supplement or nutrient it is important to do your research from a reliable source. The reason is, that just because a product has the nutrients name on the bottle, does not confirm that it came from a good source That product also requires the supporting nutrients that the main nutrient requires to be fully utilized. This is necessary to provide the desired health benefits for the body. So, in many cases, it is not enough just to take a supplement. It is how well the supplement you take is able to be utilized inside the cells to meet the needs of the body. Just because it goes in your mouth does not mean it goes into or is being used by the cells. Follow up tests should reveal a positive change. This will confirm that you are benefiting from the nutrients and supplements you are ingesting. When we take just any vitamin or supplement we may get a false sense of security, thinking we are doing what we can to be healthy. We want to take vitamins and supplements that improve our health, even if they cost more. Because there is a much higher price to pay for buying products that have zero or minimal impact on our health.

There are some people that live to eat and some that eat to live. You can have it all. There are plenty of delicious foods that can be prepared in a number of delicious ways. However, we need to know enough about food to be able to consistently have foods in our lives that have the highest health benefits. (Ref: Health Articles and Research: INTAKE #6: 18 Foods That Promote Longevity (Mercola.com)). Your journey to find and enjoy the best foods for your body is a lifelong journey. Every individual has to go on this journey to ensure they better understand, each year, the needs of their own body. It is important to know what foods make it work the best. Everyone's a little different and that's what makes a one plan fits all approach to nutrition so difficult. Over time you will find that you have developed your own plan based on what you continue to learn about your body. You will be able to confirm what works best for you by the positive changes you will experience in your health. Stick to the basics and make sure your choices are rooted in the foundations of health. Ask questions like...What have people ingested for centuries? What have people eaten or drank that have promoted health and which ones have caused health problems? Would what I drink and eat make a healthy person healthier or would it make them unhealthy over time.

In addition to us answering these important questions we must make sure our answers come from a reliable source. Sources we trust that are concerned about healthy water, food, and supplements. They should also be concerned about the methods in which the manufacturer brings these products to the store and into our homes. My most trusted source is mercola.com. I would encourage you to sign up for Dr. Mercola's newsletter. It is usually formatted for how anyone would like to consume content...video, bullet points, and full articles with research. However, you do not have to learn everything at once. You just start by gaining awareness on different topics, learning best practices, choosing and consuming better options as you learn more and more. Sometimes it is what you can add to your intake plan, sometimes it's what you want to limit or remove all together. The next step is to share good health information with your family and friends and have them share with you what they have learned so we can educate and learn from each other. This will create accountability and help everyone reach higher levels of health as efficiently as possible. We all have an easier time making healthier choices, when we are part of a group who wants the same thing for themselves and their families. Hopefully, the next generation will take what they have learned from us, add what they learn in their lifetime, and share that with their kids and friends. In hopes that a health legacy for our family's will continue to grow from generation to generation.

Foundational Habits…

Filtered Water should be the #1 fluid consumed. You will hear different things about how much water you should be drinking each day. The simplest answer is to drink half your body weight in ounces. Additional things that you need to consider with your daily water intake is any additional health concerns. Like, if you are active, or if you are going to be exposed to excessive heat. There are also things that cause dehydration, which will result in your body losing water content. So you need to be aware of how to modify these recommendations to meet your needs.

As often as you can take deep breaths of the best quality air you can .find. It can change your mental, physical, and spiritual state of mind almost immediately for the better.

Whole foods that are safely grown and come from the earth is the best place to start. Choose a wide variety of different types, shapes, and colors of whole foods. If food comes in a box, bag, or package, try to find the most natural ingredients. But, with the least number of additional unhealthy ingredients. It is proven that disease does not grow in an alkaline environment, so you can find an alkaline food chart online to make sure your shopping list includes a number of these items.

Supplements are important to ensure the body has everything it needs to function at its highest level. Any deficiencies will limit how well the body functions. Each person may have different needs based on how they eat and where they live. Take the time to intake the best variety of healthy whole foods that you can and learn what supplements would best compliment your specific needs. You can always start by taking a look at the core 4 that I mentioned above in this chapter on intake. They are a multivitamin, omega 3, probiotic, and digestive enzyme.

Chapter 3

Movement

Movement and its various forms are vital for a healthy brain and body.

Move it or lose it! Our body requires movement to be healthy. Movement helps make brains, joints, muscles, ligaments, and fascia healthy, strong, and flexible. When we consistently have movement as a foundational practice in our lives, better health is always the result. It doesn't matter where you start, just as long as you start doing something and build from there. Movement is the number one fuel source for the brain. It is required to create motion in the joints, while promoting flexibility and strength in the body.

There are a number of great exercises, exercise programs, gyms, and youtube videos that promote movement. My best recommendation is to meet the most immediate needs of your body first. Do you need to work on walking, balance, flexibility, or strength in a certain area of your body? Is there a certain activity or area of your life that is suffering because you feel weak or because of tightness and pain? Start there. When you use movement to restore health it doesn't have to look like traditional exercise. If you feel weak when getting up from sitting, practice getting stronger by getting up and down from sitting. If your legs and back are tight when you lean over to pick something up or tie your shoes and you can't touch your toes, practice getting closer to touching your toes each day. If you feel comfortable doing all your activities of daily living you can start putting movements together that will build strength, flexibility, balance, and endurance for all the other activities you enjoy doing. In order for the body to be healthy it has to move to be strong and stretched to be flexible . Your body isn't concerned if you do that in your home, the garden, the park, or at the gym. The most important thing to remember is that with movement your health will improve. This is true for every person at every age and stage of life.

When I mention movement or exercise or flexibility, people mostly focus on the muscular component. They get so focused on muscles alone that they end up damaging the joints of their body in the process. As a result, the thing that eventually stops people from doing what they love is stiffness and pain from joint problems. So, the secret to movement and being your best for a long time, is to focus on joint health first. This still includes working on muscles to be strong and flexible. However, the difference is learning how to achieve and maintain muscle health without sacrificing the health of the joints. I know the difference is subtle. Even a lot of the exercises will look the same. But being focused on posture, proper alignment, good form, and protecting the joints will help you better incorporate joint health into every movement program. Joint health utilizes joint mobility, range of motion, and engagement of supporting muscles throughout a movement. It is also important to use controlled motions throughout your movement routine. Including the process of picking up and putting down any weights you may be using. Controlled movements work the entire muscle more efficiently by keeping tension on the muscle for longer periods of time. While at the same time protecting and requiring less repetitions on the joints. This means that the muscles will get a better workout and the stress on the joints will be reduced. Protecting the joints and keeping them healthy should always be your top priority. Because, unhealthy joints are one of the greatest blind spots and pitfalls to a healthy and active life.

A person can recover rather quickly from most muscle injuries, but joint injuries can be permanent once there are bone or disc changes. This is one of the main reasons joint health deserves our attention. Joint health for the average person should not be sacrificed for one more repetition or lifting five additional pounds. It is not worth it to jeopardize the joints of your neck, shoulders, elbows, back, hips, and knees. Especially since the benefits associated with those risks are negligible for the muscles. This becomes even more apparent when you consider the increased risk and setbacks that go along with injured joints and muscles.

The best way to grow a strong foundation that you can continue to grow on, while limiting the risk of injury, is by understanding that the body needs time to adapt. Meaning you have to perform an activity long enough, like weeks or months, for your body to be prepared to handle stressing the muscles and joints at higher and higher levels. Injuries, not including falls or sudden traumas, usually occur from putting stress on a muscle or joint that has not been warmed. Injury can also occur by performing an activity at a higher intensity level than it is used too. This includes putting higher demands on muscles and joints without giving them time to adapt and grow for heavier loads. Weekend warriors can also get injured in this way as well. A lot of chronic injuries also happen on the other end of the spectrum. The person works a body part out all the time and never addresses things like rest, recovery, flexibility or range of motion of the muscles and joints. This is a bad formula for health. Eventually, over time, the joint wears down and the muscles get damaged.

So, let's talk about movement and exercise from a joint or biomechanical perspective. I hope you consider making adjustments to your movement routine that will help you make joints a priority so you can experience the difference. It was over 20 years ago that I switched from a muscle priority mindset to a joint and flexibility mindset. Just by giving joints and flexibility priority over muscle strength, and muscle strength is still important to me, I have been improving in every area of physical health. Joint health has two main components. The first component is the joint and the ligaments that hold them together. Ligaments require longer periods of time under tension (stretching) to lengthen. The extra time it takes to lengthen ligaments is worth it because on the deepest level you are actually increasing the range of motion of the joint. In addition, stretching the ligaments is also an important component for keeping space between the 2 bones that make up the joint.

This includes creating space required for the fluid and cushions that are in between the joints to protect them. The range of motion in a joint is not only important to keep joints healthy, it is also important for reducing the risk of injury. The second component are the muscles and tendons that go over joints. Muscles really enjoy protecting the joints. Joints like the protection, because it keeps them healthy. The muscles like protecting the joints because it helps them grow stronger. This is the main reason you want joints slightly bent with activity. When you stack bones and lock joints the bones and joints are doing the work. When joints are slightly bent the muscles are doing the work. This leads to much health joints and muscles. Joint health and alignment also protects muscles. The alignment of joints, align the origin and insertion points of muscles. Allowing muscles to move your body with the most power and least amount of tension and stress. This will increase muscle strength and flexibility, while reducing the risk of injury.

Our goal for taking care of our muscles is strength, flexibility, endurance, and balance. We also want to reduce the risk of scar tissue from micro or major traumas. Each day we should be unwinding tight muscles and trigger points from exercise, work, stress, and the other activities that make up our day. Unwinding tight muscles helps us to reset our muscles and set our body on a course of healing and repair. So, do your best to keep the tension and tightness on each muscle as low as possible each day. If you don't unwind muscle tension and tightness each day, tension will continue to build. This results in tightness, soreness, pain, and ultimately injury. It is always easier to care for and keep muscles healthy each day than it is to try and restore health to a muscle that has been tightening for years. Because all joints and muscles require your time and attention you may want to make a chart and rotate through all your body parts. You may, and each person usually does, have problem areas that require more attention than others. Sometimes, even when we are doing everything we can to be healthy, stress, strain, or injury in a particular area of our body can occur. It is that area that most likely deserves our time and attention most. Not to complicate things, but there are times that health problems occur due to a compensation injury. A compensation injury can be caused by an imbalance somewhere else in the body. You may require a professional to help you with those types of problems. However, taking care of yourself is never a lost endeavour, but with compensations it will be more difficult to achieve a full recovery. It may feel like no matter what you do, you are still missing something.

In general, the most important rule to follow is, spend time on your body to give it the time and attention it deserves. It will reveal what it needs to you. When you keep everything as healthy as you can, you can even unknowingly avoid compensation injuries. So, say you were to take an extra long walk or you were hiking much more than normal. In addition to warming up, stretching, and preparing for the activity. After the activity you may need to prioritize and spend some extra time on stretching your feet, ankles, calves, legs, hips, and lower back. All the muscles you used and worked during the walk or hike. It benefits your body to look at all the activities you perform in a day, even at work, in the yard, and at home from this perspective. This is what top athletes do and it keeps them performing at their best. We should be following their example and making our health the highest priority. We need to be professional athletes at the tasks we perform each day. Our health is how we make our money and it gives us the ability to enjoy our lives. So, the best way to improve the health of joints and muscles as you go through your life is to warm up the areas involved, perform the activity properly, unwind and recover tight areas when you are done that activity. Treating your activities like a professional athlete will help your joints and muscles heal longer and grow stronger.

There are a number of methods available and youtube does a great job of explaining and showing you how to get and keep the joints, ligaments, tendons, and muscles of your body healthy. The general rule is that dynamic (moving) stretches are for preparing your body for an activity. You move your body through a series of exercises and stretches that mimic the movements your joints and muscles will be performing during the activity. Static (holding one position) and Deep Stretches (holding one position for longer periods of time) are performed after an activity to lengthen muscles by holding them in a certain position for a period of time. The longer you hold the stretch the deeper the stretch. Once you have been in one stretch for 15 minutes you are at the time required to stretch the ligaments of the joints and tendons of the muscles. It is also beneficial to use muscle therapies like a trigger point stick, rolling stick, foam roller, rumble roller and all other types of massage, joint mobility, and body work. There are even exercises that are designed to lengthen and strengthen muscles at the same time. There are even many more ways of movement than I mentioned here, so try them out and find a system that works for you. The goal is to improve joint and muscle health simultaneously.

Movement (exercise, flexibility, and strength) should be done as long as you want to enjoy the many health benefits that come with them. You can not build up a big exercise health account than just coast and keep the health benefits forever. So finding activities that you enjoy, trying different activities, alternating activities, and finding different places to be active will help keep movement exciting throughout your life. People can offer movement programs for you to try that they enjoy, but it is an individual's journey to learn how and where they enjoy moving their body. Some people like the indoors, some outdoors, some like to walk, run, ride a bike, lift weights, play basketball, pickleball, yoga, karate, garden and the list goes on. When you find activities you enjoy you will feel less like you are counting the minutes and more like you are enjoying your health. Finding things you enjoy is also a great exercise in clearing your mind. (Ref: Health Articles and Research: MOVEMENT #1: The Health Benefits Of Play Time (Mercola.com)). Your body will also give you additional feedback concerning the movements it likes and dislikes. This information helps you discern which movements you should be doing, how long, and how often you should be performing them to receive the maximum health benefits. Your body knows best! We want to eliminate causing any unnecessary wear and tear on the body. This is a lifelong opportunity for health and an active life. Problems occur when you try to get healthy for a lifetime in a day, week, month, or year alone.

The best way to start a new program or activity is always to start slow, give the body time to adapt and respond to the new demands. Listen to what your body is saying so you can meet any new needs that arise. Over time you will learn how to develop and adapt programs to keep you healthy and excited about movement. Utilize professionals to learn what different options and solutions are available for you to explore. (Ref: Health Articles and Research: MOVEMENT #2: Sean Vigue Fitness Playlists (Youtube)). As you continue to develop your own special program, always listen and respond quickly to the needs of your body, the symptoms. Take care of the cause of symptoms, like stretching tight muscles, releasing trigger points, getting joints adjusted, drinking more water, and so on. These health habits will help meet the needs that the body is ultimately trying to get you to address. Symptoms are not bad, the body is highly intelligent. These symptoms are actually letting you know where a weakness exists. It provides you with all the information you need to solve health challenges and take your health to the next level.

While one workout is good and a step in the right direction. You will receive some benefits but not the full benefit of that workout. The full benefits come when you combine one workout with other workouts. You can even receive greater benefits from multiple workouts when you combine them with other complimentary habits that promote health. That one workout done 12 times, over 4 weeks multiplies the results. If you do that 144 times over a year then you get even more from each of those individual workouts. An additional multiplier is when you have other healthy habits that compliment each other like promoting LIFE with a good spine and nerve flow, INTAKE with water and good nutrition, REST, and POSITIVITY. If that isn't good enough, there is another multiplier. Your ability to have Winning Moments. Winning Moments is living your daily life in a way that minimizes any negative stresses that cause our bodies to break down from the things we do each day. While at the same time performing those same activities in a slightly different way that now promotes better health. The more we minimize the loss of health that we would need to restore, the better we can repurpose that time to produce higher levels of health. What you control, meaning, what you consistently do, how you do it, and how you spend your time will have the greatest impact on your health.

Foundational Habits…

The foundation of movement is joint health. Here is the progression for better health through movement. The first goal is to make sure all joints are moving and aligned. If not they can wear out faster. Muscle flexibility, reducing scar tissue and trigger points, releasing and remodeling fascia and ligaments is the next step. In the process we are working towards a better overall posture, while building a strong muscular system. This formula for movement will ensure that all the aspects of movement, the joints, ligaments, muscles, tendons, and fascia will be strong and healthy. This will result in limiting the risk of injury and better prepare your body to perform all the activities you enjoy. Not only now, but throughout your lifetime.

Chapter 4

Rest

Rest is when the greatest amount of healing and repair occurs in our body.

All the amazing things that happen with a good night's sleep makes rest vitally important for health. Without proper rest your body will continue to accumulate stress. This stress will have a negative effect on your body and health. This does not have to be abnormal amounts of stress. It can be normal daily stresses that we experience each and every day. Stress comes in three forms: mental, physical, and chemical. Many times all three of these types of stressors lead to similar responses in the body. These responses wear our body's down and cause damage. When the body's responses to stress stay activated for any extended period of time, and a person is not getting the proper amounts of rest, a decline in health is usually the result. Rest is the main way to give our bodies what is required to heal and repair the cells, tissues, and systems that keep us healthy and active.

When it comes to sleeping you want to do your best to prepare your body so that it can maximize its ability to heal and repair. Of all the forms of rest, sleep is proven to be one of the most important things you can do for your health. (Ref: Health Articles and Research: REST #1: How Sleep Influences Learning, Memory, And General Health (Mercola.com)). (Ref: Health Articles and Research: REST #2: Less Than 5 Hours Of Sleep Linked To Low Bone Density (Mercola.com)). Rest is also important for the health of the digestive system. Including the systems that have to work to break down food, distribute nutrients, and eliminate wastes. In order to give these systems rest, one of the best things you can do regularly is to finish your last meal of the day 3 hours before you go to bed. It is like putting those systems in neutral. This does 2 very important things. One, it helps the digestive and elimination systems rest and repair better. Second, it conserves energy from not having to process food. Now, the body can heal and repair at even a higher more efficient level. The body performs many important functions while sleeping. Like, cleaning up older and weaker cells by breaking them down. Chemicals that our body's release for healing and repair need to be able to get to the brain to tell the body to release fat to make new cells. Those healing chemicals have a problem reaching the brain when there are food components traveling through the blood. Slowing and interfering with the healing chemicals. So, we want all this healing and repair to happen more efficiently, while getting the best night's sleep. One important way we can accomplish this is by not eating 3 hours before bed. You may even notice more energy when you wake up.

Rest does not only include when you are sleeping. We need to get better at finding rest throughout the day as well. It does however take work to create environments where you can enjoy moments of rest, even in the middle of chaos. One way to improve your rest time before you go to bed, while you are sleeping, and all the next day is to prepare for tomorrow in advance. The less time you need to spend thinking about what you need to do or where you need to go tomorrow the better. You will get more rest because you are stopping your mind from racing to make decisions or remember lists. You don't want to wake you up in the middle of the night worried about what you have to do in the morning. What you don't want to forget that you have to do. What you just remembered that you have to do. Something new that you realized you have to do...have to do...have to do...have to do. Also, with your day planned you don't have to spend the entire next day trying to remember over and over again what you need to do. You reduce the chance of having to backtrack because you didn't review the entirety of the day. When you take what is on repeat in your mind and organize your day on paper or a phone it gives your mind the ability to rest. Making it possible to be more creative with the "mind" space you have made available. So now your mind has the ability to enjoy listening to a song, podcast, or book as you move through the items on your list. The sense of accomplishment that comes with checking off the items on your list helps support a positive mind.

However, here is the real test. It is important that you know your list or the order of your list usually will change. We have to be careful that these changes that are inevitable do not ruin our day. They are not always a bad thing. Life does not get in the way to where you are going, it's on the way to where you ultimately need to be. I also like the saying, life isn't happening to you, it is happening for you. The one thing I hope you would avoid with making a list is making all those things on that list only about checking boxes. This will cause you more stress if something or someone gets in the way of your list. Sometimes, in spite of a great day you may even feel disappointed because you didn't get to everything on the list. The things on your list are people, your health and things required to live and pursue your dreams, so be present and give each one your all. Relax and enjoy those moments and the moments that occur in between the boxes. Whether items on the list change or if the order changes, just keep moving forward. Go with the flow and make the most of the opportunities that each day presents.

Now I hope we have established that one of the greatest times to get rest is while we are sleeping. Providing us with better physical and mental health. However, it is also one of the most powerful times for our unconscious mind to go to work on processing the past, the present, and the future. The unconscious mind can work many times faster than our conscious mind. It supposedly has a memory of things our conscious mind has trouble recalling. Making sleep not only a time of physical healing, but also a time of processing our thoughts and experiences. This means that sleep is likely when we do our best thinking too.

There have been times when I have been working on something for hours while studying for school and my conscious mind hits a wall. As I tried to push forward things would get more and more confusing. And the harder it became to find answers. It would get so bad that I would start confusing things that I already had learned trying to find an answer. That is when I knew it was time, maybe even past the time, for me to step away and take a walk or break. Many times in that short period of rest something amazing happened. Once I put my mind on something else, my unconscious mind would kick in and I could clearly see the solution that my conscious mind was struggling to see. So, we know that the unconscious mind is powerful and works on whatever you feed it. Usually whatever you feed it last or the most. That is why it is so important before you go to sleep to monitor what you watch. You do not want things that put anxious or unwanted thoughts in your head. Also, be mindful of the type of social media content you consume before bed. Another concern about the use of cell phones before bed is that they emit a light that has been shown to disrupt sleep. Here is an article that explains how cell phone light can negatively affect getting a good night's rest. (Ref: Health Articles and Research: REST #3: How Blocking Blue Light At Night Can Help Transform Your Sleep (Mercola.com)).

Be intentional about getting your mind in a place of peace, being grateful for what you did good today, and forgiving yourself for what you wish you had done. Tomorrow is always another opportunity. There is no good reason to give yourself a hard time before you go to sleep. Sleep and a good night's rest is the next best thing you can do to prepare yourself for tomorrow. I can't stress enough the power the time before bed has on your rest and life. That is why it is a great time to feed your mind bible verses, positive affirmations, and the kind of thoughts that you want your unconscious mind to be working on through the night. This will provide us the best opportunity to get the rest and repair we need spiritually, mentally, and physically. It will prime our unconscious mind to level up to the thoughts we are feeding it. Now, when we wake up, our unconscious mind will be on track to positively impact our conscious mind. All these things together show the impact rest has on our health and life.

The most important piece of advice concerning the physical aspect of sleeping is to start with good posture and listen to your body. Sleep in positions that allow your legs to be straight, hips balanced, and spine straight. Your head and neck should be straight too. The more you keep the spine in this position the better you will support good posture. The more you have good posture the healthier the bones, discs, nerves, and muscles. The health of the spine is important to maximize healing and rest while sleeping. It is obvious that alignment is important because we all know what happens when we sleep wrong. It can cause us to have a bad night's sleep and we can even wake up sore and in pain. Utilize mattresses and pillows that support your best posture. There is no best mattress or pillow for everyone, however your body will clearly tell you which is best for you.

It is obvious how important rest is, however, it is equally important that we manage stress as well. Reducing unnecessary physical, mental, and chemical stress equals more rest. The less negative stress we have the less damage we have to repair in the first place. It is vital that we release as much stress from our day as possible, so we can heal and repair at the highest level. If we don't, stress will continue to accumulate day after day and our body's ability to heal and repair will decline. This is a bad formula. Health improves and declines over time from little choices we make each day. If we are making bad choices each day they will become little negative changes that happen over weeks and months. Those little changes will result in bigger problems over the years and decades to come. Jeopardizing our health and everything we love to do.

There are some stresses you have to address and other stresses that are a choice. The first thing to do is decide which category your stress falls under. Many stresses caused by time constraints can be reduced by better planning or leaving the house earlier. I am not trying to minimize the importance of what people stress about, just pointing out that whenever possible make sure we aren't the cause of our own stress. We also want to make sure that we are not allowing stress to snowball. Running late can turn into forgetting something, can turn into an argument, can turn into missing a turn and on it goes. However, if I don't plan, plan poorly, or get off to a late start, I try not to let it turn into a negative spiral of stress. I mentally do my best to turn everything into an opportunity. I start to look for and think about things like...What did running late protect me from? What new time schedule did this put me on that was better than the one I had planned? What can I practice and teach myself and others about being kind under stress? Where is the person I am being called to help? This can mentally help us better handle the stresses we do and the stresses we do not control. The idea is to make the most out of every situation. Use the events of your day to learn and grow. Daily stresses can be an opportunity depending on what we do with them. Stress does not always have to tear us down, turning us on ourselves and others. What is your family and friends learning from how you respond to stress and challenges? Handling stress and adapting to challenges are skills we all need to find joy in life.

Now, we all have a limit to what we can handle and we all fall short. Even when everything goes right and we are using our best tools. So, the best thing we can do when we get overwhelmed is stop and turn things around as quickly as we can instead of throwing another log on the proverbial fire. We can say we are sorry if appropriate, learn, grow, and move on. We know that negative stress can be bad for our health and should be avoided when possible. However, we also know that stress is a part of life and can help us grow. In many situations, even where people are under similar circumstances, there can be two completely different responses. One group may say that their stress or circumstances was the problem. The other group will say that their circumstances were what helped them get where they are today. They feel they would have never experienced the growth that made them who they are today if they didn't go through what they had gone through. I wrote that to say, stress has a lot to do with how we process and use it. I am not an expert and struggle with many things, but I believe so strongly in the foundations of health that I find solutions that are supported by the foundational principles in this book. Being positive and seeing life as an opportunity is congruent with those principles. Whereas other ways of dealing with stress like anger and blame do not. I am a never ending work in progress. I do my best to remain humble, educate myself, and learn from everything and everyone. I do my best to think about what I am thinking, listen to what I am listening to, and look at what I am looking at. I know my thoughts will guide how I think and feel about things. Ultimately those thoughts and feelings will determine how I act. So where I am getting my information and how I am thinking is very important to me. I want to do my part to do whatever I can to properly respond to stress. And when I fall short, over and over again, I try to get back on my feet over and over again. Sometimes an hour, day, week, or even months later. The sooner I humble myself and get help from the Lord the better. We can all use help from time to time. The brain, our past, what we see and hear each day can create a very complicated mixture of thoughts, feelings and beliefs. These thoughts, feelings and beliefs can require us to seek help. It is very important that we work through these things to be healthy. I always go to God first and those that love and serve him for help. I want to see myself as God sees me. I want to be reminded of how things really are and not what they look like. We all need to work and continue to work on our thought life. If we don't the world, disappointments, and failures will shape how we see ourselves and the world.

Chemical stresses are everywhere and growing everyday. From the way we are growing and processing food to the increase in consumption of prescribed drugs and vaccines. Plus everything else being put into our environment and bodies. So we need to always do the best we can to reduce chemical stressors. Chemical stressors are one form of stress with minimal benefits and devastating negative effects to our health. The only time chemical stressors are appropriate is for short periods of time for life saving techniques. These chemicals may be able to stabilize someone in an emergency or help fight a disease. However, it is important to know that when these chemicals are taken for extended lengths of time they have severe health risks associated with them. Many times causing more health problems than they were designed to treat. Just remember chemical stress is harmful to our body and environment. Take the time to know enough about the environment you live in. Be aware of the air you breathe, the water you drink, and the foods you eat. Always use the best products possible. Because chemical toxins can get stored in our bodies and have a negative effect on our health, avoid them whenever possible. How we handle stress will have a huge impact on our ability to get the most benefits from rest.

Foundational Habits…

All forms of rest, especially sleep, is vital for health. As I was writing this book, I continued to find one article after another promoting the health benefits of sleep. Including, how sleep reduces the risk of many health issues. This all has to do with the body's ability to heal and repair itself when given proper rest. If you do not find this chapter on sleep compelling enough to make rest a foundational principle for your health, please research it more until you do. There is no shortage of research supporting the benefits of sleep and the importance of rest to be healthy, active, and happy.

Chapter 5

Positivity

The body will achieve whatever the mind feeds it and believes.

Perspective…What perspective is true enough for you to think your best thoughts, take your boldest action, and live your greatest life. Think thoughts that make the most of your past, maximize the opportunity in front of you, and set the tone for whatever happens next. See yourself as the best version of yourself. Think the thoughts that person would think. Take the actions that person would take as if you were already that person.

We have a choice on how we see and respond to the world around us. It makes sense to make the most out of our circumstances. Start by seeing the positive in situations that you are not involved in emotionally. Because sometimes it can be harder to see the positive in things impacting you and your family. The more practice we get thinking positive thoughts, the more we will be able to have a positive response to the challenges we all encounter. We will also be an example to others on how to face challenges in a positive way. These positive thoughts over time create stronger pathways in our brain and provide us with the ability to be positive more consistently. In time, even in situations where others may find it impossible to find anything positive. In the end whatever you believe and look for you will find. No one is right or wrong, just positive or negative. Choose positivity, it is empowering, uplifting, encouraging, better for your family, friends, and health.

The health benefits of a positive mental attitude are well documented. They produce a cascade of health benefits for the entire body. Because the body will do what the brain tells it too. On the other hand, negative thoughts produce stress, which leads to disease. Interesting enough, as positive thoughts lead to healthy habits, healthy habits lead also to positive thoughts. Every time you take a walk, bike ride, swim, or exercise you feel more positive when you are done. Actually physical activity is one of the fastest ways to promote a positive environment in the body and even more positive thoughts. This is true even during those times when you feel really down. Even when you don't even feel like being active or it is the last thing you would want to do. But if you would just get started, the impact of moving the joints of the body has such an impact on the brain and nerves that it overrides many negative thoughts and feelings. I tell people that practically every time you exercise you will feel better. It is better to move your way out of negative thoughts and stress then to try and think your way out.

However, we all know that many times movement alone will not change your situation. The good news is that it can change your thoughts, then feelings, and in time your actions regarding that situation. These steps are necessary for you to play your part to change what you can and be a positive influence that others can depend on for strength. Even in situations that may never change. Excluding the things that really do matter most to us all, most things that are happening in our lives that cause us to think, feel, and act negatively are not as important or as unimportant as we make them. So, take a walk and glean a positive perspective on your situation. Focus on how you are going to use this opportunity to learn, help yourself, and others.

Positivity does not only benefit your current health status. Studies have revealed that optimism has been shown to be one of the most influential factors for longevity. (Ref: Health Articles and Research: POSITIVITY #1: Yes, Optimism Makes You Live Longer (Mercola.com)). Optimism: 1: hopefulness and confidence about the future or the successful outcome of something; 2: a doctrine that this world is the best possible world; 3: an inclination to put the most favorable construction upon actions and events or to anticipate the best possible outcome. However, longevity isn't always enough. We want those years to be healthy and active too. Optimism along with the other foundations of health, will help you live a life you can be optimistic about.

Have you ever heard that laughter is the best medicine? Well, one study on laughter found that children laugh 300 times a day on average, while adults only laugh 17 times a day. (Ref: Health Articles and Research: POSITIVITY #2: Laughter Is Good Medicine (Mercola.com)). In our family we have been accused of over laughing and thinking each other are too funny to outsiders. However, when we get together we must act like kids because we can definitely laugh 300 times a day. Laughter has made our conversations interesting and has even had the ability to bring a disagreement or fight to an abrupt end. I have seen it take people from tears to laughter at a funeral. Laughter has been the transition that can bring light into stressful situations. In those situations there may still be work left to do or pain left to deal with, but it gets enough air back in the room to breathe again.

Discipline is a key to better health. Health decisions need to be based on your goals and not on what you feel like doing or not doing. The body will not entertain and is unwavering when it comes to bargaining, reasoning, excuses, and deception. The comments and thoughts that we all need to address are "I don't have time", 'I don't feel like it", and "I can't". These thoughts can destroy your health. You may be buying these comments and the long lists of reasons you have to support them, but health and disease won't give you a break. You may even know people that are to busy too or don't like to exercise either that will support your reasoning. But your body and health will not take any of those reasons into consideration, not even for one second. Health works one way. Good habits in equals good health out and bad habits in equals bad health out over time. Many times if you can just get started all the negative feelings and excuses go away. The more you apply the foundations for health from this book, the more health you will experience, regardless of your condition or where you are starting.

There are no excuses that change these formulas for better health. So while we are on this topic, we also need to include other stumbling blocks to better health. They are "I don't know what to do" and "I can't afford it". However, probably topping the list of ways to sabotage your health is self deception..."my health is the most important thing to me." Yet it is the last thing on that persons list when considering how they spend their time and money. Many times actually spending time and money on things that have a negative affect on their health. So what is the truth? Is our health the most important thing? Can we find the 20 minutes a day our body requires to get what it needs to fuel health? Can we afford $100 a month to stay healthy and prevent many forms of chronic disease? Do we understand how expensive high insurance rates are and the cost of disease? Do we realize how much we spend on things that have a negative impact or no impact at all on our health? Money and work seem to be the most important things to us when we consider how we spend our time. Especially, when we feel healthy. It usually isn't until we lose our health that it becomes the only thing that matters. So before we lose our health in the pursuit of job titles and money, it may help to consider how our health is vital to our ability to work and make money. When people are suffering, many times they require a note to miss work. Some people have to go to work because they can't afford to miss. When you take care of your health along the way you usually don't have to make these difficult decisions. Taking care of your health allows you to have it all. Work as much as you want, make more money and feel healthy doing it. You decide when you retire and what retirement looks like. The good news is that you don't have to wait to experience the health benefits. You get to experience them all along the way, year after year.

These are not always easy questions when you are just starting out and money is tight. It takes planning and investing in yourself to get you from where you are to how you want to live the rest of your life. Think about the things that you spend money on each month and how they impact your health. Without spending any extra money on your health you can decide to buy healthier items in place of items you are already purchasing. If you decide to drink water instead of soda you can actually even save money. In the end it is truly a question of what you really value. Discipline will equal the freedom of being healthy and the freedom to do whatever you want can make you a prisoner to bad choices and disease. If you value your health, you will make healthier choices. If you value doing what you want, when you want, than that will guide your decisions. Life is usually somewhere in between the two, however the important thing is that you understand the impact of your choices over time. The last thing you want to do is make bad choices for your health and because you feel ok today. You may think the rules to health may not apply to you. This is a dangerous game to be playing.

Finding a reason that really can move you to take action is a great motivator for helping you to reach your health goals. Anyone can take care of themselves when they want to and it's fun, but what about those days that separate the pack. Those are the days that can make a big difference. They can determine if your routine keeps going or if it is coming to an end. If health alone is not enough motivation, maybe a person realizes they do not want to age like their grandparents or parents. Thinking back they remember how they never took care of one or more of these 5 foundations of health and they are suffering for it now. They may hear people saying things about how their golden years are not so golden. Other people have an activity they like so much that they do not want to lose the ability to enjoy doing what they love. There are some people who have kids or grandkids. They are caregivers and want to stay healthy and young to experience more life together with their family. I write all that to say...use whatever you can mentally to stay healthy. Better health will always benefit you. You will never be disappointed that you took care of the thing you value most, your health. This is not a selfish thing, because your health will provide you the opportunity to use it however you choose. Use it to work, play, travel, and serve others. Live unhindered by your health when following your dreams. Utilize any perspective that is true enough for you to think your greatest thoughts, take your boldest action, and live your greatest life.

Positivity and health is also linked together through our ability to be social and by the number of interactions we have with other people. It seems these social interactions have a positive impact on our health and one of the benefits is a healthier immune system. An example of this would be that your health would improve if on a consistent basis you decided to say hello to your mail man or exchange pleasantries holding a door open or with someone that is holding a door open for you. It would be nice to think that we could all be a little healthier making the world a better place.

One last comment about perspective, positivity, and optimism. While these things have been shown to promote better health, we do want to make sure that what we are believing in and hoping for are things that have true value. Meaning, the ability to deliver on our ultimate goals in life. For example, there could be a danger in being optimistic about making more money to be happier. Because making more money alone is not always associated with happiness. Especially if that optimism causes us to act contrary to who we are and what we value most. I was looking up optimism in the bible and it lead me to a story of a prosperous city who was optimistic about their wealth, but were sinning. We can put our optimism in things that don't have the ability to deliver on the promise of a better happier life. So, when I choose a perspective, positivity, and optimism I try to base them on the promises of God. I put my hope in the Lord and that has never let me down. If anything it has revealed how real God is, how true his words are, how he is in control of everything, that he is always doing what's best for us, and that he is worthy of our hope and praise.

Time with God, reading the Bible, and Prayer is the best way I have found to go through everything in life. The more consistently I rely on my time with God the better. Anytime I drift from that time with God or take it for granted like I am checking a box, I lose the joy, peace, love, comfort, mind, and thoughts that make the greatest difference in my life and the lives of others. Giving thanks, gratitude, is a powerful way to achieve a happier state of mind and positivity. (Ref: Health Articles and Research: POSITIVITY #3: Giving Thanks Does Your Body Good (Mercola.com)). Serving others is said to be one of the fastest ways to achieve happiness. It is funny how things are reversed. You would think getting what you want would lead to happiness, but it turns out being grateful and serving others, helping them get what they need, brings you even more happiness.

Foundational Habits…

Self worth and self value will guide your self talk. In each moment see and think of yourself as the best version of yourself. This image of yourself is as true as any other image you could be holding onto. The only difference is that it is free of negative thoughts, what negative things people have said to you, disappointments from your past, and learning experiences that you may have labeled as failures. Your self worth, self value, and self talk need to be positive for you to be healthy mentally and physically. Choose positivity to show respect for your past, maximize your present, and set the course for your future.

Chapter 6

The 5 Foundations of Health

There are questions that science will always be trying to answer, bottle, and sell to us. However, health has followed the same rules for centuries. No matter what position science seems to take, it always comes back to the proven time tested methods on how to achieve better health. They may find new ways to utilize these principles for better, faster results. But in the end, following these principles over time will always lead to better health. The best news is that they work no matter where you are starting from or what you are going through. These principles of health do not guarantee that you never have a symptom or have to live with a disease. What they do guarantee is that you will be the healthiest version of yourself. This will allow you to live your best life, no matter what life has in store for you.

This book is about the foundations of health that apply to everyone. These 5 Foundations Life, Intake, Movement, Rest, and Positivity are perfectly designed to work with how our bodies are designed. Every cell will work based on the environment that you create for it. If its needs are met it will be the best cell. If the needs of the cell are not met it does not have the ability to work at its best or support the tissue it is a part of and so on. That goes for every cell. The cell does eventually get older and need to be replaced by a new cell. The quality of the "new" cell will be determined by the present environment you have created. This environment not only determines how the new cell is created, it also influences how the cell functions throughout its life cycle. The majority of this environment and consequently the health of new cells are determined by these 5 foundational principles. Over time trillions and trillions of cells will be replaced. As a result, how you address these 5 principles consistently over time will determine the health of your cells and ultimately your body. These changes to the cells impact how you feel, what you can and can't do, your ability to enjoy life, and how you live it.

Now, there is an age old question of nature vs. nurture. Is it the genes or the choices that people make that have a bigger impact on their health over time. We would all have to say that genetics clearly plays a role, like when you look at a child and they look exactly like a parent or in the case of twins. However, there have been studies on twins that show their health can vary, even for identical twins. One of the most important advances in genetics has been the study of epigenetics. Epigenetics is how all our genes are affected by the choices we make. Those include all our choices, even positive or negative thoughts. Because our thoughts actually change the physiology of our body. This is evident by the negative impact on health that occurs with mental stress.

So, what epigenetics says is that just because we have certain genes, that does not mean those genes are always on or off. What researchers have discovered is that it is the choices we make and the environments or physiology those choices create in our body that actually turn on and off genes. While bad choices can turn on unhealthy genes and turn off healthy genes, good choices can turn on healthy genes and turn off unhealthy ones. These choices that turn on and off genes determine how our genes influence our health. It is the science where nature and nurture blend together. In the end it is in our best interest that we be accountable and empowered, for the sake of our health, to focus on what we do control. We have the ability to make healthy choices by following the principles of Life, Intake, Movement, Rest, and Positivity. These gene studies confirm that these choices will positively or negatively impact our genes and our health. Just think about that, what we do control has been determined to actually influence what we once thought we couldn't control, our genetics.

Nature's rules apply to all creation and the number one rule is to live by nature's rules. Like when a garden gets less water than it needs, leaves begin to droop. At this point there is still time to give the plant what it requires to not only survive, but to recover, thrive, and produce at its best. Now, if we ignore or do not stay in tune with the needs of the garden it will struggle to flourish. In addition, the garden's needs can change with the amount of sun, rain, or heat and it is our job to be aware and make adjustments concerning how different circumstances can change those needs. If it gets a little water, but still less than it needs, it may look a little better, but it will still be missing what it requires to produce at its best. In the end the fruits or vegetables that the garden produces will tell a lot about the health and life of that garden. The better we are able to provide the garden with its foundational requirements like water, sunlight, and soil, the better they will flourish. Our body is the same way. A healthy, active life, and the ability to fight disease are indicators of how well we are meeting the foundational needs of our body.

Of all the foundational principles, LIFE through spinal joint health, is my number one priority. I found that protecting my brain and nerves is the best plan for a long healthy active life. The life impulses that run through the brain and nerves which are protected by the joints of the spine impact how our body does everything. Including intake, with things like digestion, transportation of nutrients, and elimination of wastes, just to name a few things. Movement, with how the body moves and feels throughout a person's life. In addition to how long the joints last, based on the care they have received through the years. And, it is even difficult to get a good night's rest and stay positive with pain in joints irritating your muscles and nerves. These are some of the many reasons why I prioritize life through joint health. My muscles can still be very important to me and healthy without sacrificing the spine or joints. The spine and joints do not have the same ability to recover as muscles. So to exercise for muscles alone, at the cost of the spine or joints is too high a cost. Arthritis and disc changes are unlikely to reverse easily and can be the cause of unnecessary suffering. There are ways of exercising muscles while protecting the spine and joints. It is a subtle difference, but vitally important. There aren't many people that end up missing out on life or are suffering because they lift less weight than someone else. It is usually because they have chronic joint issues from not making joint health a priority in their life. It isn't their fault, I never knew, and I suffered for it. Millions of other people are suffering and their families' will continue to suffer until we help them. To be healthy everyone needs to learn the importance of joint health and how to keep joints healthy. Joint health, including spinal health, is important for the health of the brain and nerves. This is the main reason why it is vitally important that we know how to take care of the joints of the spine from birth through every age and stage of life.

My other book Winning Moments focuses on how to turn everything you normally do in a day into better health. I thought this was extremely important because I had figured out a way to solve two of people's biggest problems. Finding the time to take care of themselves and money. One of the main goals of the book was to eliminate poor daily habits that lead to injury and poor health. The other main goal was to perform those same exact activities in a way that could promote better health. All we had to do was show people how to properly perform daily activities as if they were doing it as their workout. A great example of Winning Moments is a person who sits a lot in a car, at work or home. You can improve this person's health just by showing them how to sit properly and the different exercises they can do while sitting. They can learn how to sit longer while working out their core and feel better at the end of the day. Instead of sitting improperly and injuring their back. Winning Moments is full of examples like this and can be used as a daily road map for better health.

These 5 Foundations of Health together with Winning Moments will lead to better health for everyone. However, each person has needs that are unique to them. We have to learn about and listen to our body concerning the best ways and times to meet those needs. If we do, we will maximize and support how our body works, grows, and produces health in our lives. This includes our ability to be active and age normally. We can learn how others are caring for their health by watching and speaking to them, but it is most important that we find what works best for us.

Investing in our health is an ongoing process. I am continually learning new things about health, trying different things on my own and observing what others are doing. I want to continue providing my body with the best opportunities available for better health. Working on movement may involve exploring or expanding on spinal mobility, flexibility, strength, or soft tissue work. It also includes all the other foundations of health as well. Like, how I am eating or reviewing what I am reading, watching, and listening too. It may be looking at what time I go to bed, especially if I notice I am getting up later and later and missing out on my morning routine. Sometimes it is learning something new and sometimes it is getting back to good habits that have gotten lost over time. It is important to remember that it is not always about adding to your health routine, sometimes its' reducing or eliminating activities that don't work for you. Your body type may not be a good fit for certain types of exercise or certain foods may not benefit your digestive system. This could be the case for people with food allergies or sensitivities. It's possible to also experience great health benefits from removing or minimizing negative health routines, like over training, which may have been put in place unintentionally as a way to cope with stress.

The most important thing is that you take the time to find what works best for you and the things you enjoy. You can take the time to build up your health account, but if you stop it won't take long to spend what's left in the account. You may have to write a big check unexpectedly. How would you feel if you woke up and nothing was left in your account? Especially when you need it the most. So, to be safe, never stop investing in your health. Find things you enjoy, continue to build up your health and have fun along the way. This road map to health will provide you with many treasures on the way to your best life.

Try not to be over concerned about the perfect program, just be concerned about progress. You will learn so much along the way. Much more than if you never get started. It is not about doing everything all at once, it is just about doing something. Each day, miraculously, things will begin to come together more and more.

Chapter 7

My Story

I thought health was how I looked and felt, I loved to exercise, and worked at gyms. I would work out for hours each day and I loved to play basketball. I was doing everything I knew and had been taught to make me healthy. I was exercising and eating right. Unknowingly, at the same time I was destroying my spine and discs, while damaging my nerve system. You see, nobody told me how to take care of my spine. That's a big reason I want to make sure I help as many people as possible learn how to take care of their spine and teach it to their family and others. I want to help people not only avoid the suffering I had to go through, but now I know they need a healthy spine to live their best life.

The pain and discomfort I experienced was so bad that I went and had surgery. No one ever told me that there were any other options. Following the surgery, I had relief, but 2 years later I started to have the same pain again, fortunately, it was at that time that I learned about chiropractic care. That's when I learned how to care for my spine, discs, and nerve system as a foundation of health. Surgery had cut away the damage to my spine , but it did not remove what caused damage, which was a subluxation. Subluxation is a chiropractic term for a spinal joint that has lost motion and causes irritation to the spine, discs, and nerves. It is also the cause of spinal arthritis and many disc diseases, like degenerative disc disease. Once I started caring for the subluxation and focusing on spinal joint health with a chiropractic adjustment schedule my health has been improving ever since. Chiropractic has also taught me to focus on the best ways to perform everything I do, even the littlest things. In addition I keep a checklist of habits I want to perform each day that helps me to live the foundations of health. I have a desire to continually improve my health, especially the health of my spine. I have had such great success with this formula for health in my life and the life of those under my care, that I want to share it with as many people, family's, and generations as possible. This book is what I have learned from more than 20 years of experience. Some of my first lessons were how to live with excruciating pain, which lead me to learn about the power of chiropractic care. Now, I've learned how to live a healthier more active life without pain, beyond exercise and eating healthy alone. The same foundational principles I have learned and used to get out of pain, I have found to be the same principles that allow my health to continue to improve each day. LIFE, INTAKE, MOVEMENT, REST, POSITIVITY! These principles can do the same for you.

You may not need life, intake, movement, rest, positivity...sleep, water, good nutrition, strength, flexibility, endurance, balance, good posture, chiropractic care, soft tissue work, massage, acupuncture, physical therapy, yoga, dental work, yearly exams, blood work...to feel good, but your body needs them to be healthy.

I want to thank Jennifer, my wife, and daughter, Makenzie. We have things we love to do together and watching me obsess about being healthy may not be one of them, but you created the space for me to be me, so I say...THANK YOU!

Thank you to my parents…true fitness fanatics...I have many great memories of going to gyms, playing basketball, racquetball, doing aerobics, taking bike rides, runs, long hikes, and walks together. You guys are still going strong. I'm so glad we have a legacy of health to share with each other. I am grateful for the time and quality of life, treasures, that these foundations of health have provided for us.

Health Articles and Research

An interactive guide to great articles and research for better health.

Use the url link or camera on your phone to scan the QR codes(make sure in your phone settings, under camera, scan the QR codes option is on, if the camera is not reading the codes, or get a QR code scanner app)

INTRODUCTION
- #1: 10 Ways To Live Longer (Mercola.com).......................................
  https://articles.mercola.com/sites/articles/archive/2019/12/24/10-ways-to-live-longer.aspx

LIFE
- #1: The Nervous System In 9 Minutes (CTE Skills.com on youtube)....
  https://www.youtube.com/watch?v=44B0ms3XPKU

- #2: Structure Of The Vertebral Column - Functions Of The Spine - Bones Of The Vertebrae (Whats Up Dude on YouTube).......................
  https://www.youtube.com/watch?v=lzSJBlt8m6U

- #3: Stiffness And Pain In The Morning And After Activity (FreshStartChiro1 on YouTube)..

  https://youtu.be/45m_pCYPNPjk

INTAKE

- #1: Water Poisoning Alerts Hidden From Public (Mercola.com)..........

  https://articles.mercola.com/sites/articles/archive/2019/10/09/legionnaires-disease-in-drinking-water.aspx?utm_source=dnl&utm_medium=email&utm_content=art1HL&utm_campaign=20191009Z1&et_cid=DM363552&et_rid=725271213

- #2: What Makes Most Foods So Dangerous, Even "Healthy Foods" (Mercola.com)...

  https://articles.mercola.com/sites/articles/archive/2019/10/01/toxicity-in-food.aspx?utm_source=dnl&utm_medium=email&utm_content=art1HL&utm_campaign=20191001Z1&et_cid=DM358597&et_rid=719641600

- #3: The Truth About Sugar Addiction (Mercola.com)............................ https://articles.mercola.com/sugar-addiction.aspx

- #4: How Gut Bacteria Influence Your Metabolism (Mercola.com)......... https://articles.mercola.com/sites/articles/archive/2019/09/30/gut-bacteria-and-metabolism.aspx?utm_source=dnl&utm_medium=email&utm_content=art1HL&utm_campaign=20190930Z1&et_cid=DM367399&et_rid=718992236

- #5: Vitamin D Resource Page (Mercola.com)...................................... https://www.mercola.com/article/vitamin-d-resources.htm

- #6: 18 Foods That Promote Longevity (Mercola.com)........................... https://articles.mercola.com/sites/articles/archive/2016/01/04/foods-for-longevity.aspx

MOVEMENT

- #1: The Health Benefits Of Play Time (Mercola.com)............................
  https://articles.mercola.com/sites/articles/archive/2019/12/14/the-power-of-play-documentary.aspx

- #2: Sean Vigue Fitness Playlists (Youtube)...
  https://www.youtube.com/user/motleyfitness/playlists

REST

- #1: How Sleep Influences Learning, Memory, And General Health (Mercola.com)...
  https://articles.mercola.com/sites/articles/archive/2019/03/30/health-benefits-of-sleep.aspx

- #2: Less Than 5 Hours Of Sleep Linked To Low Bone Density (Mercola.com)...

https://articles.mercola.com/sites/articles/archive/2019/12/12/sleep-bone-density.aspx

- #3: How Blocking Blue Light At Night Can Help Transform Your Sleep (Mercola.com)..
https://articles.mercola.com/sites/articles/archive/2016/05/05/blocking-blue-light.aspx

POSITIVITY

- #1: Yes, Optimism Makes You Live Longer (Mercola.com)...................
https://articles.mercola.com/sites/articles/archive/2017/01/12/optimism-promotes-longevity.aspx

- #2: Laughter Is Good Medicine (Mercola.com)....................................
https://articles.mercola.com/sites/articles/archive/2019/10/03/laughter-therapy.aspx?utm_source=dnl&utm_medium=email&utm_content=art1HL&utm_campaign=20191003Z1&et_cid=DM358617&et_rid=721100849

- #3: Giving Thanks Does Your Body Good (Mercola.com).....................

  https://articles.mercola.com/sites/articles/archive/2019/11/28/effects-of-gratitude-on-health.aspx

www.ingramcontent.com/pod-product-compliance
Lightning Source LLC
Chambersburg PA
CBHW020622220526
45463CB00006B/2646